Sinusitis Diet Guide

A 5-Step Plan to Manage Congestion Triggers and Support Allergy Season (With Sample Meal Plans and Recipes)

mf

Disclaimer

This guide is provided for informational and educational purposes only and should not be interpreted as medical, nutritional, or professional advice. The author is not a licensed physician, nurse, dietitian, or mental health provider. Reading this guide does not establish a patient–provider relationship of any kind.

Always seek the guidance of a qualified healthcare professional before starting, changing, or discontinuing any supplement, diet, or lifestyle program. If you are pregnant, breastfeeding, managing a chronic medical condition, or taking prescription medications, consult your physician or pharmacist before considering any product mentioned in this guide.

The author and publisher make no representations or warranties regarding accuracy, applicability, fitness, or completeness of the information contained herein. While every effort has been made to ensure scientific accuracy and currency, medical knowledge and research evolve continually. Readers are responsible for verifying information and making decisions in consultation with licensed professionals.

Use of this guide and any information contained within it is at your own risk. The author and publisher disclaim all liability for any loss, injury, or adverse outcome that may result from the use or misuse of this material.

No supplement, diet, or practice discussed in this text is intended to diagnose, treat, cure, or prevent any disease. No outcomes or benefits are guaranteed.

Product names, supplement formulations, diet frameworks, and trademarks mentioned are the property of their respective owners and are used for identification only. Any images or illustrations that appear in related materials are licensed stock or educational placeholders.

Table of Contents

Introduction

Sinus problems are an all-too-common challenge, especially for those who battle recurring congestion, facial pressure, and lingering discomfort. These symptoms often become more pronounced during certain times of year, particularly when allergens like pollen are at their peak.

For many people, sinus symptoms also seem to worsen after eating particular foods or meals a frustrating pattern that can disrupt daily life and make even simple tasks feel burdensome. Recurrent or chronic sinusitis doesn't just cause localized discomfort; it can sap your energy, interrupt your sleep, make breathing feel like a chore, and erode your overall productivity and quality of life.

That's why targeted dietary management is more than just a lifestyle tweak; it's an important and effective strategy for anyone seeking reliable, long-term sinus relief. While there are pharmaceutical treatments and even surgical options for managing sinusitis, many individuals find that making specific changes to their everyday eating habits can provide significant relief. Your daily food choices have a direct impact on inflammation, immune response, and the body's ability to recover from or resist sinus issues.

This Sinusitis Diet Guide is designed to give you a clear, actionable plan for identifying and managing the dietary triggers that may be contributing to your sinus symptoms. Following this stepwise program, you'll learn how to break the cycle of congestion and support your sinus health through practical day-to-day meal and grocery planning. The focus here is not on complex medical procedures or in-depth immunological theories, but on what you have the power to change every single day: your food choices, eating habits, and nutritional routines.

In this guide, you will discover:

- What sinusitis is, including the most common causes and symptoms
- How sinusitis develops and why it becomes chronic or recurrent for some people
- The most common dietary triggers for sinus congestion and inflammation
- A proven 5-step dietary plan to help identify and manage your personal food triggers
- Detailed food lists highlighting what to eat and what to avoid to reduce sinus symptoms
- Practical tools for tracking your symptoms and dietary choices, so you can troubleshoot and measure your progress

- Sample meal plans and easy-to-follow recipes designed to make implementation realistic, sustainable, and enjoyable

Throughout, you'll find foundational explanations to help you understand your condition better, as well as practical strategies you can start using right away. These include tips for reading food labels, shopping smart, and planning ahead so you're never caught off guard by hidden triggers. You'll also find troubleshooting advice for those times when symptoms flare up despite your best efforts, along with encouragement and guidance to help you stay motivated and consistent as you adopt new habits.

By the end of this guide, you'll be equipped not only with knowledge but also with a concrete plan and the tools you need to take control of your sinus health. Whether you're newly diagnosed or have struggled with sinusitis for years, these dietary strategies offer a pathway toward lasting relief and improved well-being.

What Is Sinusitis? Symptoms, Causes, and Risk Factors

Sinusitis, often simply called a sinus infection, is a condition that affects millions of people worldwide, causing discomfort, fatigue, and disruptions to everyday life. Understanding the basics of sinusitis including its types, hallmark symptoms, primary causes, and risk factors is an essential first step before exploring how dietary changes can assist in symptom management and prevention.

Clinical Definition of Sinusitis

Sinusitis is the inflammation or swelling of the tissue lining the sinuses' hollow cavities located within the skull around the nose and eyes. Healthy sinuses are filled with air, but when they become blocked and filled with fluid, germs can grow and cause an infection. The defining feature of sinusitis is this inflammation, which leads to a range of uncomfortable symptoms and can significantly impact quality of life.

Sinusitis is typically classified into two main categories, based on the duration and frequency of symptoms:

1. **Acute Sinusitis:**
    - Characterized by a sudden onset of symptoms.
    - Usually lasts up to four weeks.
    - Often follows a cold or upper respiratory infection.
2. **Chronic Sinusitis:**
    - Symptoms persist for 12 weeks or longer, despite attempts at treatment.
    - May involve repeated or ongoing episodes, sometimes with less obvious acute symptoms.
    - Chronic cases can lead to thickened sinus lining, persistent congestion, and long-term discomfort.

These two forms may share similar symptoms, but chronic sinusitis is generally considered more resistant to standard therapies and is more likely to require a holistic approach, including dietary management for lasting relief.

Symptom Checklist: Recognizing Sinusitis

Whether acute or chronic, sinusitis is most commonly recognized by a cluster of symptoms that can range from mild to severe. The following checklist can help you identify possible signs of sinusitis:

- ***Facial Pain or Pressure***: A feeling of tightness, pain, or fullness in the cheeks, forehead, or between/behind the eyes is very common.

- ***Nasal Congestion***: Blockage or stuffiness in one or both nostrils, making it difficult to breathe through the nose.
- ***Thick Nasal Discharge***: Mucus may become thick, yellow, or green, and can drain from the nose or down the back of the throat (postnasal drip).
- ***Reduced Sense of Smell and Taste***: Many people notice that smells and flavors become less distinct.
- ***Headache***: Pressure changes within the sinuses can translate into headache, especially upon waking or when bending forward.
- ***Fatigue***: Persistent or recurrent sinusitis often leads to general tiredness due to poor sleep and chronic discomfort.
- ***Tooth or Upper Jaw Pain***: Discomfort may radiate to the teeth or upper jaw.
- ***Ear Pressure or Fullness***: Some may experience a sensation of ear fullness or even mild hearing changes.

Chronic sinusitis may also contribute to persistent bad breath, cough (often worse at night), and, in some instances, mild fever.

Understanding these symptoms and noting their frequency and severity is a critical beginning as you navigate dietary and lifestyle modifications. Early identification often leads to better, more sustainable management outcomes.

Underlying Causes of Sinusitis

The reasons why someone develops sinusitis are varied, and sometimes more than one factor is at play. Below are the core causes that set the stage for sinus inflammation:

- ***Infections***: Viral infections (such as the common cold) are the most frequent triggers for acute sinusitis. Bacterial infections may follow if the initial illness does not resolve, while fungal infections are rarer but can affect those with weakened immune systems.
- ***Allergens***: Environmental allergens like pollen, animal dander, dust mites, and certain molds can irritate sinus linings, especially during peak allergy seasons. Repeated exposure may lead to ongoing inflammation and chronic symptoms.
- ***Structural Blockages***: Deviated nasal septum, nasal polyps, or other anatomical variations can impede normal drainage from the sinuses, creating an environment for inflammation and persistent infection.
- ***Environmental Irritants***: Exposure to cigarette smoke, intense air pollution, strong odors (like those from chemical cleaners or perfumes), or occupational dusts can irritate the delicate mucosal lining of the sinuses and promote inflammation.
- ***Other Contributors***: Swelling in the nasal passageways from frequent colds, changes in air

pressure (e.g., during air travel), and even some dental problems can also lead to sinusitis.

A clear view of the root cause of your symptoms can offer major benefits, as it helps you identify the most effective paths to relief through medical care as well as lifestyle or dietary choices.

Risk Factors: Who Is Most Susceptible?

Certain people are more likely than others to develop sinusitis, and knowing your personal risk profile allows for more targeted preventive strategies. The most significant risk factors include:

- ***Allergies***: Individuals with hay fever (allergic rhinitis) or other sensitivities to environmental allergens experience sinus inflammation more easily, especially during certain times of the year.
- ***Frequent Respiratory Infections***: Having repeated colds, flu, or other upper respiratory tract infections raises the risk of developing both acute and chronic sinusitis, as the sinuses are repeatedly exposed to pathogens and inflammation.
- ***Smoking and Passive Smoke Exposure***: Tobacco smoke irritates the respiratory tract, decreasing natural defenses and making it easier for sinuses to become infected and inflamed.

- ***Anatomical Variations***: Birth defects, injury-induced nasal passage abnormalities, or growth of polyps can all impede sinus drainage, setting up the conditions for recurrent or lingering infections.
- ***Immune System Deficiencies***: Those with impaired immune function due to illness or medication—are at higher risk of infections, including fungal sinusitis.

Other factors such as exposure to severe air pollution, working in environments with high levels of dust/chemicals, and having untreated allergies or asthma may also increase your vulnerability.

Symptom-Tracking Log: Establishing Your Personal Baseline

A cornerstone of effective dietary change for sinusitis management is being able to track and correlate symptoms with potential triggers. Keeping a dedicated symptom-tracking log doesn't just enhance communication with your healthcare team, it empowers you to notice connections between food, environment, and how you feel day to day.

Below is a simple template you can use as a starting point. Update it daily or whenever symptoms change noticeably:

Table 1: Sample Symptom-Tracking Log

Date	Main Symptoms (Check all that apply)	Severity (1-5)	Notable Foods Eaten	Environ mental Factors	Medica-tions Used
	□ Facial pressure/ pain				
	□ Nasal congestion				
	□ Discharge/ postnasal drip				
	□ Fatigue				
	□ Reduced smell/taste				
	□ Other: ___________				

<u>Tips for Using the Log:</u>

- Mark symptoms each day and rate the severity (1 = very mild, 5 = severe).
- Note specific foods, drinks, or new products consumed around the time of symptom changes.
- Track environmental exposures such as the presence of pets, pollen counts, or smoking.
- Adjust as needed: Add notes on sleep quality or emotional stress for a fuller picture.
- Keep your log easily accessible, such as in a daily planner, notes app, or dedicated journal.

This data builds a valuable baseline for future dietary modifications, helping you recognize both obvious and subtle trends over time.

A clear grasp of sinusitis, its symptoms, causes, and personal risk factors gives you the knowledge needed to make informed decisions as you begin the Sinusitis Diet 5-Step Plan outlined in the coming chapters. This foundation helps you identify what to change, monitor progress, and tailor your approach for effective, lasting sinus relief.

Food-Related Sinus Congestion Triggers (Fundamentals)

When it comes to managing sinusitis, dietary triggers are often overlooked contributors to ongoing inflammation, congestion, and discomfort. Emerging research and clinical observation confirm that certain foods and food groups can provoke or worsen sinus symptoms, especially during allergy season or in those with chronic sinus issues.

Awareness of these triggers and the mechanisms behind them allows you to take meaningful action through dietary changes and serves as the foundation of the Sinusitis Diet 5-Step Plan presented in later chapters.

Checklist of High-Probability Dietary Triggers

Not all foods are created equal when it comes to their impact on sinus congestion and inflammation. Research and patient feedback consistently highlight a set of high-probability dietary culprits. Below is a focused checklist of foods most likely to aggravate sinusitis symptoms for sensitive individuals:

- ***Dairy Products***: Milk, cheese, yogurt, ice cream, and similar items are frequent offenders. Dairy can thicken mucus, increase overall mucus production, and promote obstructive congestion in some people with sinusitis, especially when consumed in large quantities or during active allergy phases.
- ***Gluten-Containing Grains***: Wheat, barley, and rye may worsen inflammation for individuals with gluten sensitivity or intolerance. While not universally problematic, a subset of people notice fewer sinus symptoms after removing or reducing gluten-containing foods from their diets.
- ***Refined Sugars***: Sweets, pastries, soda, and other foods high in added sugar have pro-inflammatory properties and may disrupt immune function, contributing to sinus swelling or heightened susceptibility to infections.
- ***Processed Foods***: Packaged meals, fast foods, and snacks commonly contain a mix of preservatives, unhealthy fats, and additives that can trigger or sustain inflammation and exacerbate sinus congestion.
- ***Alcohol***: Wine, beer, and spirits are known to act as vasodilators and mucosal irritants. Alcohol can dehydrate the body, increase nasal stuffiness, and

stimulate allergic-like reactions or flushing, making sinus symptoms more pronounced.

Starting with this checklist, you can focus your observation and elimination trials on foods with the highest likelihood of contributing to your symptoms.

Mechanisms of Trigger-Induced Inflammation and Mucus Production

Food-related sinus congestion is not the result of a single process, but rather a cascade of events triggered in susceptible individuals. Several mechanisms explain how dietary triggers can aggravate sinus symptoms:

1. ***Mucus Production and Thickness***: Foods like dairy may stimulate glands in the upper respiratory tract to produce thicker and more abundant mucus. This excess mucus can clog sinus passages, leading to the familiar sensation of pressure and stuffiness.
2. ***Immune Activation and Inflammatory Response***: Ingestion of certain proteins (such as those in wheat or cow's milk) can prompt immune reactions in people with sensitivities, resulting in localized swelling and congestion. Chronic exposure to these triggers keeps the immune system in a "heightened" state, promoting persistent inflammation.
3. ***Exacerbation of Allergic Pathways***: Some foods may cross-react with environmental allergens or trigger

histamine release, intensifying symptoms in allergy-prone individuals during peak seasons.

4. ***Dehydration and Mucosal Drying***: Alcohol and overly salty processed foods dehydrate the mucosal surfaces, making them more susceptible to irritation and less effective at clearing out pathogens and allergens.

The cumulative result is swelling, blockage, and difficulty clearing mucus, which can perpetuate or intensify sinusitis symptoms.

Comparison Table: Immediate vs. Delayed Food Sensitivity Reactions

Pinpointing whether a food is causing your sinus symptoms can be confusing. Some triggers elicit rapid reactions, while others cause issues only hours or days later. Understanding this distinction can help you match symptom patterns to their dietary sources.

Table 2: Comparison Table

Type of Reaction	Onset After Eating	Common Symptoms	Typical Examples
Immediate Food Sensitivity	Within minutes to 2 hours	Nasal stuffiness, runny nose	Dairy, alcohol, some preservatives
		sneezing, throat irritation	artificial colorings
Delayed Food Sensitivity	4 hours to 72 hours	Gradual congestion, fatigue	Gluten-containing grains, refined sugars

		worsening chronic sinus symptoms	processed foods

Immediate reactions are often easier to spot, occurring shortly after exposure. Delayed reactions require careful tracking, as symptoms can build insidiously over time and may not be linked to a single meal. This is where a structured symptom and food diary becomes an invaluable tool.

Failure Modes: Misattribution and Underestimation

Two of the most common barriers to successful dietary management of sinusitis are failing to identify food triggers and underestimating the effect of seemingly minor exposures.

1. ***Misattribution of Symptoms***

   It's easy to assume that all sinus symptoms stem from infections or environmental allergens. Many people do not consider dietary causes, especially when symptoms overlap with cold, flu, or allergy manifestations. For instance, a congestion flare-up may be blamed on seasonal pollen counts when, in reality, it coincides with increased dairy or alcohol intake.

2. ***Underestimating Cumulative Effects***

   Repeated small exposures to problematic foods such as a splash of milk in coffee every morning or the occasional sweet treat can have a cumulative effect.

Even if a single serving does not cause a dramatic reaction, ongoing low-level exposure keeps the sinuses in a state of chronic irritation, preventing full recovery. This underlines the importance of a thorough and sometimes strict elimination trial when assessing food involvement in sinus congestion.

Decision Criteria Chart for Justified Elimination Trials

Not everyone needs to eliminate every highlight food from the checklist. The goal is to target your personal triggers based on observed patterns and response to removal. Use the following decision criteria chart to determine when a justified elimination trial is warranted:

Table 3: Decision Criteria Chart

Condition	Recommended Action
Sinus symptoms (congestion, pain, etc.) recur or worsen shortly after consuming a specific food or drink	Begin an immediate elimination trial for that item.
Symptoms gradually worsen with no clear environmental trigger and intake of suspect foods is regular	Conduct a 2-4 week elimination of high-probability foods (dairy, gluten, processed foods, sugars, alcohol).
Multiple suspected triggers, with overlapping symptoms and delayed responses	Apply a phased elimination—remove all probable triggers, then reintroduce one at a time to evaluate effects.
Inconclusive patterns after journaling and environmental adjustments	Seek professional evaluation (nutritional or allergist referral) for further assessment.

Careful documentation during the elimination period is crucial. Monitor daily for improvement in congestion, energy levels, and secondary symptoms (headaches, fatigue, postnasal drip). Positive results especially with re-challenge (adding the food back and observing return of symptoms) strongly implicate the food as a trigger.

Building Confidence for Step 3: Identifying Your Unique Combination

Those new to food-based sinusitis management often ask, "How do I know if I'm on the right track?" Building confidence starts with a structured, patient approach:

- Use your symptom-tracking log daily, cross-referencing symptoms with foods eaten.
- Prioritize high-probability triggers during elimination, but remain alert to other foods that repeatedly coincide with symptom flare-ups.
- Only make one dietary change at a time during reintroduction for clearer results.
- If progress is unclear, consider a professional assessment to identify less common or hidden dietary irritants.

Remember that while food is a significant factor in many chronic sinusitis cases, allergies, environmental exposures, and structural factors should never be entirely discounted.

With a strong understanding of food-related sinus congestion triggers and a strategy for identifying your personal sensitivities you are poised to explore the Sinusitis Diet 5-Step Plan. The next chapter will introduce this action-oriented approach, providing stepwise guidance for real-world, sustainable sinus relief.

The Sinusitis Diet 5-Step Plan: Overview and Ruleset

Taking control of sinusitis often requires more than just identifying triggers; it calls for a systematic, actionable plan to address sinus issues at the source. The Sinusitis Diet 5-Step Plan offers exactly that: a phased, evidence-grounded strategy to manage food-related congestion triggers, support sinus recovery, and build long-term resilience during allergy season and beyond. This approach provides a clear path for progression, allowing you to personalize every phase to your unique needs while maximizing your chances for lasting sinus relief.

The 5-Step Phased Approach for Sinusitis Dietary Management

This stepwise framework was developed in response to the complexity and individuality of sinus triggers. Rather than a "one-size-fits-all" elimination, the plan is designed to help you discover, remove, and ultimately adapt to your personal sinus congestion sources all while maintaining nutrition and quality of life.

The phases are as follows:

1. Identify (Step 1)
2. Eliminate (Step 2)
3. Substitute (Step 3)
4. Support (Step 4)
5. Maintain (Step 5)

Each phase is supported by specific actions, with diagnostic checklists empowering you to know exactly when and how to proceed to the next step.

Step Definitions: What Each Phase Means and Why It Matters

Step 1: Identify

The first phase lays the groundwork: observing and systematically pinpointing foods most likely to aggravate your sinus symptoms. This process involves keeping a food and symptom journal, referencing typical trigger lists (dairy, gluten, refined sugars, processed foods, and alcohol), and tracking both immediate and delayed symptom patterns. Success here requires honesty and consistency identifying even seemingly minor contributors is crucial for progress.

Step 2: Eliminate

Once likely triggers are identified, the next step is a structured elimination. You will remove high-probability sinus offenders from your diet for a defined period typically 2-4 weeks to allow inflammation to subside and to assess whether symptoms improve. The elimination phase is best approached with commitment and complete avoidance, as even small exposures can sustain congestion and block meaningful improvement.

Step 3: Substitute

Elimination alone isn't sustainable or healthy without suitable replacements. The substitution phase is your opportunity to find nutrient-rich, hypoallergenic alternatives for eliminated foods. This could mean choosing plant-based milk or gluten-free grains instead of wheat, or focusing on whole, unprocessed foods over commercial snacks. Optimizing substitutes helps ensure you maintain variety, adequate nutrition, and culinary enjoyment despite restrictions.

Step 4: Support

Here, you focus on building a sinus-friendly dietary foundation for healing and immune support. Add foods rich in anti-inflammatory nutrients think leafy greens, oily fish, turmeric, ginger, berries and optimize hydration. Prioritize meals and snacks that minimize mucus production and support ongoing sinus health, especially in the lead-up to or during allergy season.

Step 5: Maintain

The final phase transitions your short-term changes into sustainable, long-term habits. Maintenance means reintroducing previously eliminated foods one at a time (if desired), tracking your body's response, and establishing an accountability structure whether through self-monitoring, digital tools, or routine check-ins. Adaptation to social situations, travel, or unexpected exposures also becomes a focus.

Diagnostic Checklist: When and How to Progress

Knowing when to move from one phase to the next is essential for maximizing relief and minimizing risk of relapse. The following diagnostic checklist will help you monitor progress and make informed decisions throughout your sinusitis diet journey:

Identify → Eliminate

- You have at least one food or drink that consistently precedes symptom onset or worsening in your journals.
- Patterns suggest a link between certain foods and congestion, energy dips, or pressure, not otherwise explained by environmental triggers.

Eliminate → Substitute

- After 2-4 weeks of strict elimination, you've noticed improvement in key symptoms (less congestion, easier breathing, reduced facial pain, improved energy).
- You are struggling to maintain variety, nutrition, or satisfaction on your current plan and need safe alternatives.

Substitute → Support

- You are able to sustain your new eating habits but want to further accelerate recovery and boost immune resilience.
- Ongoing sinus symptoms have significantly reduced, but you want to minimize the risk of setbacks during allergy or peak infection seasons.

Support → Maintain

- You've established a core set of anti-inflammatory meals and snacks you enjoy.
- Sinus symptoms are consistently low or absent; you can function normally and wish to test food reintroduction, or maintain your new habits long-term.

Examples of Transition Markers and Milestones

Many readers ask: "What changes should I expect, and when is it safe to advance?" While every individual differs, transition markers and milestones help you judge readiness for the next phase:

- ***Symptom Resolution Timeline***: Initial improvements in congestion and energy may appear within 1-2 weeks of trigger elimination, especially for obvious foods like dairy and alcohol. More insidious triggers such as gluten or processed foods may require up to 4 weeks for benefits to become clear.
- ***Reintroduction Tolerance Levels***: Reintroduce one eliminated food at a time after a symptom-free baseline is achieved. A food that provokes congestion, fatigue, or "sinus fullness" within 72 hours is likely an ongoing trigger and should be avoided longer term. If tolerated with no symptom return, reintroduce the next food.
- ***Plateau Phases***: If you experience a plateau with no further symptom reduction despite elimination, it is possible that a non-dietary factor or overlooked subtle trigger is at play. In such cases, consider refining your journal, reviewing less common triggers, or consulting a professional.

5-Step Plan At-A-Glance: Action Framework

For clarity and daily use, the following framework summarizes the 5-Step Plan in one view:

1. **Identify**
    - Track every meal, snack, and beverage alongside symptoms.
    - Use the high-probability trigger list and note any temporal correlations.

2. **Eliminate**
    - Remove all identified likely sinusitis triggers for 2–4 weeks.
    - Commit to 100% avoidance for the trial period.
    - Monitor changes daily, looking for symptom relief.

3. **Substitute**
    - Replace eliminated foods with nutrient-dense, low-reactivity alternatives.
    - Keep meals balanced: protein, healthy fats, whole grains, and abundant non-starchy vegetables.
    - Watch for accidental exposures and hidden ingredients.

4. **Support**
    - Prioritize foods high in vitamin C, zinc, quercetin, and omega-3s.
    - Stay hydrated with water, herbal teas, and broths.
    - Prepare meals ahead to reduce temptation and exposure to processed foods.

5. **Maintain**
    - Gradually reintroduce individual foods and track effects.
    - Adjust plans for events, travel, or seasonal fluctuations (e.g., during spring and fall pollen peaks).
    - Use tracking tools and support groups as needed for accountability.

This action framework gives you a stepwise map to reliably reduce—or even resolve—sinusitis-related symptoms by leveraging dietary choices.

Table 4: Summary Table: The 5 Steps and Their Purpose

Step	**Purpose**	**Key Action**	**When to Transition**
Identify	Pinpoint likely dietary triggers	Keep food/symptom journal	Consistent patterns observed
Eliminate	Remove triggers to allow healing	2–4 weeks total avoidance	Noticeable symptom reduction
Substitute	Maintain nutrition and satisfaction	Swap triggers with safe foods	Diet is balanced, symptoms stable
Support	Bolster healing and resilience	Optimize anti-inflammatory intake	Symptoms consistently low/absent
Maintain	Cement habits, test reintroduc-tion	Gradual, monitored reintros	New foods tolerated, stable sinus health

Set Your Expectations

It is common to feel impatient or overwhelmed at the outset. However, real and lasting improvements in sinus congestion and quality of life are achievable with this phased, patient approach. Small setbacks are normal. Treat each phase as an opportunity for learning, not just as a set of rules to follow.

In the next chapters, you'll find detailed instructions for each step complete with tracking tools, food lists, and troubleshooting advice to help guide you toward clearer breathing and better overall health.

Following this structured, evidence-informed approach, you set yourself up for clearer breathing, fewer flare-ups, and more confidence in managing sinusitis with every meal.

Step 1—Identify Problem Foods (Mechanisms)

In tackling sinusitis through dietary changes, the cornerstone is accurate identification of the foods most likely to trigger or worsen congestion, swelling, and discomfort. Step 1 of the Sinusitis Diet 5-Step Plan is where dietary detective work begins: it's about creating a clear, evidence-based map between what you eat and how your sinuses respond. This chapter provides you with hands-on tools, practical decision criteria, and technology options to transform vague dietary suspicions into actionable strategy.

Why Identification First?

Sinusitis is complex and its triggers vary not only person-to-person, but sometimes for the same person in changing seasons or circumstances. Foods that reliably worsen symptoms for one person may not affect another at all. Therefore, a methodical approach is necessary to avoid both unnecessary dietary restriction and missed triggers.

The Role of Food Journaling: Building Your Self-Assessment Toolkit

Central to Step 1 is meticulous food journaling. A well-kept record lets you spot trends, identify connections, and document what might otherwise be forgotten. This is more than just noting what you eat; it's a daily log that features:

- The exact foods and drinks consumed (ingredients, brands, preparation)
- Time of consumption
- Onset, duration, and severity of sinus symptoms (congestion, pressure, headache)
- Additional environmental or life factors (pollen count, stress levels, travel, medication use)

To facilitate this, start with a dedicated food journaling worksheet. You can print a template or use a lined notebook with columns for date, time, foods eaten, symptoms (scored, for example, 0–10), and notes about anything unusual. Commit to recording everything for at least two weeks even minor snacks and seasonings.

Table 5: Sample Food Journaling Worksheet Template

Date	Time	Food/ Beverage	Portion/ Brand	Symptoms (0-10)	Notes
4/10	8am	Oatmeal (w/ milk)	1 cup, Brand X	3 (congestion)	Used honey
4/10	10am	Coffee (black)	1 cup	3	
4/10	12pm	Turkey sandwich (white bread, tomato, lettuce, mayo)	1 sandwich	7 (pressure)	Mild head-ache

Completeness and honesty are crucial. Even foods you consider 'innocent' or 'healthy' can occasionally be triggers, so nothing should be overlooked in this process.

Symptom Timeline Correlation: Pinning Down Potential Irritants

Sinus reactions to foods are not always immediate. Some provoke symptoms within an hour (such as dairy for some people), while others may take 12–72 hours for congestion or facial pressure to manifest. Capturing this timeline is pivotal for narrowing down suspects.

To link exposure to reaction more precisely, employ a symptom timeline correlation table. This table helps you "plot" foods against when symptoms arise:

Table 6: Sample Symptom Timeline Correlation Table

Day	Food Consumed	Time of Consumption	Symptom Onset	Symptom Details
1	Ice cream	7 pm	Next morning	Blocked nose, facial pressure
2	Pasta (wheat)	12 pm	Evening	Mild congestion
3	Chicken stir-fry (no known triggers)	6 pm	No symptoms	—

Over several days, such patterns become clearer. This correlation is important for both "classic" quick reactions and insidious, delayed effects especially from foods like gluten, processed snacks, or certain additives.

Using Elimination and Re-Challenge as Diagnostic Tools

Once your journaling points to likely trigger foods, the elimination-and-re-challenge method becomes a rigorous next step. Here's how to proceed:

1. ***Eliminate***: Remove all suspect foods from your diet completely for a trial period (usually 2–4 weeks). Use your worksheet to ensure none are consumed, even in small amounts or hidden forms.
2. ***Observe***: Monitor and record daily symptoms. Note any improvement in congestion, sinus pressure, frequency/severity of flare-ups, and general wellness.

3. ***Re-Challenge***: Once symptoms have stabilized or improved, reintroduce only ONE food at a time. Eat a reasonable portion (ideally twice in one day), then observe and journal for 72 hours.
4. ***Result***: If symptoms recur, that food is a "primary suspect" and should remain excluded for now. If there is no reaction, it can likely be safely included in your diet again.

The cycle of elimination and re-challenge ensures you are not indefinitely avoiding foods that aren't true triggers, while reliably pinning down your high-impact culprits.

Assessment Criteria: Ranking Food Suspects

During this investigative phase, it helps to create a ranking system for food suspects:

<u>Primary Suspects:</u>

- Foods that consistently precede sinus symptom onset or worsening (within 72 hours)
- Typical triggers identified by research and clinical reports: dairy, gluten, refined sugars, processed meats, and alcohol.
- Foods with clear and repeated timeline correlations during your journal period

<u>Secondary Suspects:</u>

- Foods that may be infrequent, less clearly linked, or potentially problematic only in combination with others
- Items associated with possible delayed, low-grade symptoms or only noticed under certain circumstances (e.g., during allergy seasons, when stressed, or in combination with alcohol)

Keep a running table, listing offenders and your confidence rating (e.g., "high evidence" vs. "possible"). Tackle primary suspects first during elimination. This stepwise method keeps the process both manageable and evidence-based.

Digital Tracking Tools and Mobile Apps for Streamlined Food-Symptom Mapping

While traditional pen-and-paper journaling is effective, digital solutions can enhance accuracy and make data review far more efficient. Today, several apps allow you to log foods, symptoms, and triggers with ease. Key features to look for include:

- Customizable food and symptom entries
- Time-stamped logs
- Reminders to enter meals or symptoms throughout the day
- Data export options for sharing with healthcare professionals

Some widely used app options include food diary apps (like MyFitnessPal, Cara Care, Symple), as well as condition-specific trackers that allow multi-symptom correlation. Select an app that lets you customize symptom fields essential for capturing sinus-specific patterns and that can export your data for backup or deeper analysis.

With digital tracking tools, you can quickly see patterns such as daily or weekly symptom peaks, which makes it much easier to identify chronic offenders over time.

Best Practices for Step 1

Here are key success strategies for the identification phase of your Sinusitis Diet Plan:

- ***Start at a "baseline"***: If possible, begin journaling when you are at your most typical state (neither in a major flare nor during acute illness).
- ***Be thorough***: Record everything, including beverages, condiments, and "just a bite" snacks.
- ***Check for combinations***: Some people react only when certain foods are eaten together (e.g., dairy plus sugar, or bread with processed meat).
- ***Consider context***: Record environmental conditions (high pollen days, exposure to smoke, or increased stress), as these can confound results.

- ***Revisit and reflect***: Review your food and symptom logs weekly to look for connections you may not notice day-to-day.

The hardest part of Step 1 is often sticking with it and not glossing over "cheats" or assuming you know a food's effects. Remember, the more consistently and accurately you journal, the faster you'll move from vague frustration to clear answer and ultimately, sustained sinus relief.

Once you've collected 2–3 weeks of thorough data and identified your prime suspects, you're ready to transition to the Elimination phase (Step 2). This structured move is covered in the next chapter, including details on avoidance, substitution, and tracking symptom changes.

At the core of the sinusitis diet approach is empowerment through self-observation. Identifying your dietary triggers doesn't just offer symptom relief; it builds confidence in your body's feedback and offers strategies for adaptation in future allergy seasons.

Achieving Step 1 means you now possess the most effective tool for lasting sinus relief: personalized, evidence-based insight into your unique triggers. Keep tracking, reviewing, and making informed choices based on your own data this will set you up for the targeted, transformative actions in the next phases of your Sinusitis Diet journey.

Step 2—Eliminate and Substitute Sinus-Triggering Foods (Execution)

Once you have identified your personal dietary triggers by carefully tracking foods and symptom patterns, it's time to move into the elimination and substitution phase. This step is where real transformation takes place: not only do you systematically remove likely offenders from your meals, but you rebuild your kitchen and dietary habits with effective, delicious alternatives that keep sinus congestion and flare-ups at bay.

Elimination Phase Protocol: Duration and Strictness

The elimination phase is designed to give your body a clean break from foods most likely to provoke sinus-related inflammation, excess mucus production, or congestion. To be effective, the elimination phase demands both strictness and adequate time. For maximum clarity:

- ***Remove all identified or suspected trigger foods*** from your diet for a minimum of two weeks four weeks is optimal if chronic sinusitis symptoms have been long-standing or severe.
- ***"Strict avoidance" means reading every food label***, asking about ingredients when eating out, avoiding "may contain" or cross-contaminated foods, and not consuming even small amounts. Even minor exposure can cause lingering or recurring symptoms, muddying your results.
- ***Keep logging your meals and daily symptoms*** as before; this data becomes essential for confirming improvement and planning reintroductions later.

Key targets for elimination typically include dairy products, gluten-containing grains, refined sugars, highly processed foods, and alcohol, as these are among the most common dietary triggers in sinusitis sufferers. However, your personal list should always come from your previous tracking.

Substitution Checklist: Allergy-Friendly and Low-Inflammation Alternatives

Elimination may sound restrictive, but the key to long-term dietary change is finding satisfying, practical substitutes for every eliminated trigger. Substitution prevents feelings of deprivation and also ensures nutritional balance. Below is a checklist to guide your choices:

- ***Milk and Dairy Products***: Use plant-based milks (such as oat, almond, or coconut), coconut yogurt, and dairy-free cheeses made from cashews or soy.
- ***Gluten-Containing Grains***: Swap with naturally gluten-free options like quinoa, brown rice, buckwheat, millet, or certified gluten-free oats.
- ***Refined Sugar***: Satisfy sweetness with modest portions of fruit, unsweetened applesauce, or natural sweeteners such as stevia or monk fruit.
- ***Processed Foods***: Opt for homemade meals and snacks using whole-food ingredients; use olive oil, herbs, and spices to season.
- ***Alcohol***: If removing alcohol, substitute with sparkling water, herbal teas, or "mocktails" using citrus, berries, or ginger for flavor.
- ***Allergenic Additives***: Replace commercial sauces and dressings with simple homemade blends—think olive oil and lemon, or tahini and garlic.

Aim for nutrient-dense replacements, prioritizing anti-inflammatory foods like leafy greens, berries, turmeric, sweet potato, salmon, and pumpkin seeds whenever possible.

Decision Tree: Detecting and Preventing Accidental Exposure

Accidental exposure is a top reason why elimination phases fail to yield clear results. To help you guard against mistakes, use the following practical decision tree when planning, preparing, and eating food:

1. Is this a home-cooked meal using whole, single-ingredient foods?
   - ☐ Yes: Proceed, ensuring all staple ingredients are on your "safe" list.
   - ☐ No: Go to next step.
2. For packaged foods, have you read every bit of the ingredient label—including fine print about allergens, "processed in a facility," and additives?
   - ☐ Yes: If trigger-free, it's safe.
   - ☐ No: Do not consume, set aside until you can verify.
3. Eating out or ordering in did you ask about all ingredients, including sauces, thickeners, and "hidden" components?
   - ☐ Yes: Assess based on staff's knowledge and willingness to accommodate.
   - ☐ No: Avoid, or choose a menu option you can fully verify.
4. Are you in a situation where food sharing or buffet-style serving could lead to cross-contamination?
   - ☐ Yes: Either serve yourself first with clean utensils or bring your own meal/snack.

If at any point you cannot verify the contents or preparation process, it is safest to avoid that food during the elimination window. When clarity is your goal, "when in doubt, leave it out" is a sound rule.

Common Pitfall Index: Cross-Contamination & Hidden Ingredient Sources

Several pitfalls can undermine even the most dedicated efforts to avoid sinus triggers. Being aware of these risks will keep your results (and progress) on track:

- ***Shared Toasters, Pots, and Utensils***: Gluten, dairy, or processed food residues can linger on shared cooking equipment. Always use designated tools or thoroughly clean before use.
- ***Sauces, Marinades, and Dressings***: Many commercial products include milk solids, gluten (as thickeners), artificial colors, or flavor enhancers. Opt for homemade or trusted brands with full disclosure.
- ***Pre-Prepared Deli Meats and Meat Alternatives***: These often contain nitrites, gluten-based fillers, or "natural flavors" that may be allergenic or inflammatory.
- ***Snack Foods and Candy***: Even simple items (like potato chips or dark chocolate) can harbor dairy, gluten, soy, or trace amounts of processed additives.
- ***Restaurant Meals Labeled "Free-From"***: Mislabeling and kitchen cross-contact happen frequently. Always

question preparation techniques and ingredient sourcing.

- ***Drinks***: Alcohol, flavored coffees, and even smoothies may contain hidden syrups, creamers, or sweetener blends.

Combatting these pitfalls requires vigilance but also planning. Prepare "safe" snacks for travel, double-check labels often, and err on the side of caution during the elimination phase.

Pantry Overhaul Checklist: Setting Up a Trigger-Free Kitchen

To support your elimination journey, it's essential to create an environment where safe choices are easy and accessible. Use this comprehensive pantry overhaul checklist:

- ***Remove or box up all items containing your target triggers***: store them out of sight to minimize temptation or accidental use.
- ***Restock with whole foods***: fresh or frozen fruit and vegetables, plain meats and fish, legumes, gluten-free grains, and safe oils (like extra virgin olive, avocado, or coconut).
- ***Replace condiments with minimally-processed or homemade versions***: mustard, vinegar, and fresh herbs, for example.
- ***Label all new pantry staples*** with "safe" stickers for quick identification during meal prep.

- ***Purchase containers to separate allergen-free*** flours, grains, and snacks from those for other household members.
- ***Keep a shopping list*** of reliable go-to brands and products that fit your elimination and substitution criteria.
- ***Organize a dedicated shelf or section*** for "elimination phase" items so meal planning feels streamlined.

A kitchen and pantry set up in this way does more than guard against hidden triggers; it also greatly reduces stress and decision fatigue. When safe options stay visible and easy to reach, consistent adherence becomes far easier.

Troubleshooting and Reinforcement

During the elimination period, some people may experience accidental lapses or realize a food is embedded in a less obvious product. If this occurs, don't be discouraged; simply resume strict avoidance and note the event in your tracking log. If symptoms flare, document carefully. Consistency improves results, but a single lapse isn't a failure persistence is key.

Supporting Family or Shared Spaces

If you live with others who do not require the elimination diet, communicate your plan and ask for support in shared kitchen spaces. Labeling, using dedicated utensils, and having a separate area for your foods helps to prevent mix-ups and makes food prep less stressful for everyone involved.

Step 2 of the Sinusitis Diet Plan requires both commitment and strategic action. A rigid, well-planned elimination paired with nourishing, anti-inflammatory substitutes maximizes your chances of revealing true food-symptom connections and feeling measurable relief. Setting up a safe environment, anticipating pitfalls, and building a pantry you trust are the most powerful tools for ensuring a successful elimination phase.

Your next step will be to focus on choices that actively support sinus and immune wellness, further solidifying the improvements gained by removing your most problematic foods. Continue tracking, stay organized, and celebrate your progress as you feel clearer, breathe easier, and regain energy for the things you love.

Step 3—Support Sinus Wellness through Nutrient-Rich Choices

After eliminating and substituting sinus-triggering foods, your next milestone in the Sinusitis Diet 5-Step Plan is to actively support healing and defense by prioritizing nutrient-rich, anti-inflammatory choices. This step moves beyond "what not to eat" and into strategic eating, choosing foods and nutrients that foster clear sinuses, thin mucus, and support robust immunity.

This chapter provides both the rationale and practical guidance you need, focusing on key vitamins, minerals, and plant-based nutrients, shopping strategies, hydration, macronutrient balance, and meal preparation for sustainable sinus health.

Table of Vitamins, Minerals, and Phytonutrients Linked to Sinus and Immune Health

Certain nutrients possess properties that directly or indirectly support sinus health. Incorporating them on a daily basis is essential for those seeking to reduce congestion, support immune response, and maintain healthy sinus tissue. Below is an at-a-glance table organized by function:

Table 7: Nutrients and Their Function

Nutrient	Role in Sinus/ Immune Health	Food Sources
Vitamin C	Antioxidant; supports immune defense; may reduce histamine response	Citrus fruits, kiwi, berries, bell peppers
Vitamin A	Maintains mucosal linings; supports immunity	Sweet potatoes, carrots, spinach
Vitamin E	Antioxidant; supports epithelial repair	Sunflower seeds, almonds, avocados
Zinc	Modulates immunity; supports wound healing	Pumpkin seeds, chickpeas, lentils
Selenium	Antioxidant; assists detoxification	Brazil nuts, mushrooms, eggs
Omega-3 Fatty Acids	Reduce inflammation; support tissue integrity	Oily fish (salmon, mackerel), flaxseed, walnuts
Quercetin (phytonutrient)	Natural antihistamine; antioxidant	Red onions, apples, capers, kale
Curcumin (from turmeric)	Anti-inflammatory, supports immune health	Turmeric spice
Bromelain (enzyme)	Reduces mucus, aids in nasal drainage	Pineapple

Aiming for variety ensures that you cover all supportive nutrients and maximize synergy among them.

Example Shopping List for Anti-Inflammatory Foods

Building a practical, anti-inflammatory grocery list makes it easier to translate theory into daily habits. Here's a sample cart for your next shopping trip, tailored to sinus and immune health:

- *Leafy greens*: Spinach, kale, arugula, Swiss chard
- *Cruciferous vegetables*: Broccoli, cauliflower, Brussels sprouts
- *Berries*: Blueberries, strawberries, blackberries
- *Oily fish*: Salmon, sardines, mackerel (wild-caught, if possible)
- *Nuts and seeds*: Pumpkin seeds, chia seeds, flaxseeds, walnuts
- *Citrus fruits*: Oranges, grapefruit, lemons
- *Roots and tubers*: Sweet potato, carrots, beets
- *Allium vegetables*: Red onions, garlic, scallions
- *Fresh ginger and turmeric root*
- *Legumes*: Chickpeas, lentils, black beans
- *Fresh herbs*: Parsley, cilantro, basil
- *Extra virgin olive oil* (for salads and gentle sautéing)
- *Plant-based milk alternatives* (unsweetened, for those who avoid dairy)

A well-stocked kitchen with these items creates a strong base for meals that combat inflammation and support healthy sinus drainage.

Hydration Tracker and Fluids Selection Chart for Optimal Mucus Thinning

Proper hydration is one of the simplest, yet most overlooked, dietary tools for sinus health. Water helps thin mucus, making it less sticky and easier to drain from the sinus passages. For people with sinusitis, inadequate fluid intake can quickly worsen congestion.

Set a daily goal of at least 8 cups (2 liters) of total fluids, increasing intake during periods of illness, allergy flare-ups, or high heat. Use this chart to diversify your hydrating options:

Table 8: Hydration Tracker and Fluids Selection Chart

Fluid	Sinus Health Benefits	Tips for Use
Plain water	Directly thins mucus	Sip throughout the day
Herbal teas (ginger, peppermint, chamomile)	Anti-inflammatory, soothing	Serve hot for additional steam benefit
Diluted fruit infusions	Flavorful, encourages drinking	Add slices of citrus, berries, or cucumber to water
Broths (vegetable or bone)	Hydrates, delivers minerals	Use as a base for soups/stews
Coconut water	Contains electrolytes	Choose unsweetened; limit to 1 cup/day

Limit caffeinated or sweetened beverages, which can be dehydrating or promote inflammation. Monitor your hydration with a simple app or notepad, aiming for pale yellow urine as a reliable indicator of adequate intake.

Framework for Balancing Macronutrients to Stabilize Blood Sugar and Limit Inflammation

Stable blood sugar plays a key yet often overlooked role in control of inflammation and, by extension, sinus congestion. Sharp rises and drops in blood glucose can worsen inflammatory activity, especially when meals contain high amounts of refined carbohydrates or added sugars.

Use the following framework to balance your macronutrients at every meal:

- ***Carbohydrates***: Choose slow-digesting, fiber-rich sources such as quinoa, sweet potato, brown rice, lentils, or vegetables.
- ***Proteins***: Lean poultry, fish, legumes, or tofu deliver building blocks for immune cells and tissue repair.
- ***Fats***: Favor anti-inflammatory fats like olive oil, avocado, walnuts, and limited portions of cold-water fish.
- ***Plate method***: Fill half your plate with non-starchy vegetables, one-quarter with protein, and one-quarter with starches or whole grains.

Minimize or avoid processed snacks, bakery items, and hidden sugars these substances fuel inflammatory responses and can worsen symptom severity. Pairing each meal with protein and fiber slows sugar absorption, reduces energy crashes, and promotes better resilience against sinus flare-ups.

Meal-Prep Guide for Building Nutrient-Dense Breakfasts, Lunches, and Dinners

Sustaining dietary changes is easier when you have a repeatable system for preparing meals in advance. Use these meal-prep strategies to lock in sinus-friendly nutrition all week:

Breakfast Ideas:

- Overnight oats with blueberries, flaxseed, and a splash of plant-based milk
- Spinach and red onion omelet, topped with avocado and fresh herbs
- Chia pudding with diced kiwi, pumpkin seeds, and a dash of turmeric

Lunch Options:

- Quinoa salad with kale, chickpeas, diced bell pepper, and lemon-olive oil dressing
- Lentil soup with carrots, celery, garlic, and sliced turmeric root

- Grilled wild salmon over arugula, with roasted sweet potatoes and steamed broccoli

Dinner Combinations:

- Baked mackerel or trout with sautéed Swiss chard, and a side of beets
- Vegetable stir-fry (broccoli, snow peas, red onion) with tofu and ginger-turmeric sauce, served with brown rice
- Stuffed bell peppers with black beans, tomatoes, and fresh cilantro

Tips for Successful Meal Prep:

- Batch-cook grains and legumes at the start of the week for easy assembly.
- Pre-wash and chop leafy greens and vegetables for salad bases or quick sautés.
- Roast root vegetables in large quantities; store in airtight containers for fast reheating.
- Prepare homemade vinaigrettes using olive oil, lemon juice, and fresh herbs.
- Portion nuts, seeds, and berries as ready-to-eat snacks.

Having key components on hand helps reduce daily decision fatigue and ensures each meal actively supports sinus relief and overall vitality. Step 3 centers on empowering your body to heal, defend, and restore itself through intentional nutrition.

Focus on nutrient-dense, hydrating, and anti-inflammatory foods, and incorporate practical prep strategies to create a foundation for lasting sinus health and fewer congestion episodes during allergy season and beyond.

Step 4—Allergy Season Adaptation Plan

Seasonal allergies can sharply undermine progress for anyone managing sinusitis with dietary strategies. When pollens and molds proliferate, your immune system is already on high alert, making it more vulnerable to aggravation by certain foods.

Instead of waiting for symptoms to flare, a proactive approach tailoring your diet in anticipation of allergy season can be a powerful defense for maintaining clear sinuses and reducing discomfort. Step 4 in the Sinusitis Diet 5-Step Plan is designed to help you adapt your meal plan and food choices ahead of and throughout peak allergy months.

Timeline for Dietary Adjustments in Peak Pollen and Mold Seasons

Allergy seasons are dictated by local environmental factors, primarily the types and levels of airborne pollens (tree, grass, weed) and molds. Many people with sinusitis notice intensifying congestion, facial pressure, and postnasal drip as pollen counts rise. For best results, begin dietary adaptations at least 2-3 weeks before your region's forecasted peak pollen or mold counts. This grants your body time to lower its baseline inflammation levels and build up resilience.

Adopting an allergen-aware eating plan involves:

- Checking local pollen or mold forecasts (see below for lookup guide) in late winter or early spring for spring pollen, summer for grass pollen, and late summer to autumn for ragweed and molds.
- Intensifying anti-inflammatory meal choices before and during peak counts; focus on foods rich in vitamin C, quercetin, and omega-3s that support your immune system and help modulate allergic reactions.
- Avoiding food triggers that typically cause congestion such as dairy, gluten, refined sugars, and highly processed foods for the entire allergy window, not just after symptoms start.

If you are especially sensitive, consider ongoing dietary vigilance through the full allergy season, only relaxing restrictions once daily pollen counts return to baseline.

Decision Criteria for Temporary Elimination or Increased Restriction

During times of heightened allergy risk, even foods you tolerate at other times of year may contribute to worsening symptoms. Use these criteria to decide when to implement or tighten eliminations:

- ***Your history***: If your symptoms spiked in previous allergy seasons despite dietary efforts, consider stricter avoidance of all known culprits (dairy, gluten, processed/packaged foods, excess sugars, and alcohol) throughout peak months.
- ***Pollen/mold forecast***: If your local index predicts counts in the "moderate" or "high" category, temporarily remove even borderline foods or those you've only partially reintroduced post-elimination.
- ***Symptom log***: Escalate your elimination strategy if you notice early warning signs such as increased sneezing, runny nose, facial pressure, or tiredness even if you haven't reached "full" allergy season.
- ***Other factors***: Recent illness, stress, or exposure to smoke and pollutants increase your reactivity threshold. Be extra strict during these periods.

Adapting your plan means you may scale back to a more extensive elimination (removing all top triggers and questionable foods) during high-risk intervals, then gradually reintroduce foods as environmental exposures wane. This cyclical, responsive elimination not only reduces flare potential but also helps you clarify which foods are truly problematic year-round.

Local Pollen Index Lookup Guide for Personalized Planning

Personalizing your adaptation plan hinges on timely awareness of local conditions. Use these steps to stay one step ahead:

1. Identify reputable pollen and mold forecast services (such as your regional weather provider, local allergy clinics, or dedicated pollen tracking websites).
2. Set calendar reminders to check pollen/mold forecasts weekly in the lead-up to expected high seasons, and daily during peak months.
3. Track your city or ZIP code; pollen loads can vary dramatically over short distances.
4. Note which kinds of pollen trigger your symptoms most (trees, grass, weeds), and adjust your timeline accordingly.

Pair this external data with your own symptom log. If you notice that congestion starts 2-3 days after pollen counts rise, move your dietary adjustments even earlier the following season. This personalized "seasonal map" forms the backbone of your Allergy Season Adaptation Plan, helping you act preventively instead of reactively.

Examples of Anti-Allergy Food Combos and Immune-Boosting Snacks

Food can be more than just fuel; during allergy season, your meals and snacks should work synergistically to modulate inflammation and protect your airways. Prioritize anti-allergy nutrients and combinations that stabilize immune response and support sinus health:

- ***Fresh pineapple and ginger smoothie***: Rich in bromelain (an enzyme that helps thin mucus) and ginger (with natural anti-inflammatory properties).
- ***Sliced red apples with pumpkin seeds***: Apples contain quercetin, a plant compound shown to have natural antihistamine effects, while pumpkin seeds deliver immune-boosting zinc.
- ***Roasted sweet potato, beet, and kale salad***: A powerhouse mix providing vitamins A and C plus beta-carotene and minerals that strengthen mucous membranes.
- ***Wild-caught salmon or sardine salad wraps***: Omega-3 fatty acids curb allergy-driven inflammation, while leafy wraps add vitamin K and fiber to ease digestion and absorption of nutrients.
- ***Turmeric-spiced lentil and spinach soup***: Curcumin in turmeric is a potent anti-inflammatory, and lentils provide plant-based protein for immune repair.

<u>For on-the-go snacking:</u>

- Sliced orange or kiwi fruit (vitamin C)
- Handful of unsalted walnuts (omega-3s)
- Carrot and celery sticks with hummus (quercetin, antibacterial effect of garlic)
- Homemade trail mix with sunflower seeds, dried berries, and chopped Brazil nuts

Adopt these as grab-and-go snacks or meal additions, especially before outdoor exposure or on high-pollen days. This not only reduces the risk of flare-ups, but also ensures your body is primed to handle environmental insults.

Seasonal Adaptation Checklist and Calendar Template

Building repeatable routines makes allergy season preparation less daunting. Use the following checklist and incorporate a calendar template for seamless execution:

Pre-Season (2–3 weeks before forecasted increase):

- Check local pollen/mold forecasts and set up alerts.
- Review previous year's symptom logs to identify early warning trends.
- Eliminate top triggers: dairy, gluten, excess sugar, processed foods, and alcohol.
- Stock pantry with anti-inflammatory staples (citrus, berries, greens, nuts, oily fish, legumes, fresh herbs).

- Prepare small batches of immune-boosting snacks to keep available throughout the week.

During Peak Season:

- Continue monitoring forecasts daily and updating your elimination/substitution plan as needed.
- Keep hydrated and drink at least 8 cups of water or anti-inflammatory herbal teas per day.
- Prepare or portion out anti-allergy food combos for each day.
- Eat fresh or lightly cooked vegetables at every meal.
- Limit outdoor activities when pollen counts are highest (midday); shower and change clothes after returning indoors.

Post-Season (as local counts normalize):

- Gradually reintroduce low-risk foods one at a time, tracking symptoms closely.
- Reflect and record which strategies were most effective for next year's plan.
- Meet with your health provider or nutritionist as needed to refine your approach.

Table 9: Sample Calendar Template for Allergy Adaptation

Month/ Week	Forecast	Actions to Take	Symptom Notes
Week 1 (March)	Pollen low	Begin eliminating known triggers	

Week 2 (March)	Pollen rising	Introduce anti-inflammatory snacks	
Week 3 (March)	Moderate pollen	Step up hydration, batch-cook meals	Early congestion?
Week 4 (March-April)	High pollen	Full elimination, avoid eating out	Log daily symptoms
May	Pollen down	Begin gradual reintroduction	Monitor reaction

Fill in your region's critical months and append your own notes to adapt this template to your personal environment and allergy patterns. Completing this process annually ensures that short-term inconveniences are outweighed by long-term relief and symptom control.

Step 5—Long-Term Maintenance and Sustainable Habits

Relief from sinusitis symptoms through dietary changes marks only the first part of the process; maintaining these improvements over months and years requires new habits, practical tools, and consistent support. Step 5 of the Sinusitis Diet 5-Step Plan guides you to establish daily routines, safely expand your food choices, handle social situations, set up accountability systems, and maintain a symptom-free life. Incorporating these strategies into your lifestyle makes long-term sinus health both achievable and sustainable.

Habit Tracker Template for Routine Incorporation of Beneficial Dietary Practices

Consistency is essential for lasting results. Without regular attention to food choices, it's easy to slip back into old routines that once triggered your sinus issues. A structured habit tracker enables you to convert positive intentions into actual daily practices and gives you early warning when consistency begins to drift.

Use a habit tracker template designed for sinusitis management, capturing these key domains:

- Daily intake of sinus-friendly vegetables (at least one serving of leafy greens and one vitamin C-rich food)
- Hydration (targeting 8 or more cups of water or herbal teas per day)
- Complete avoidance of major triggers (dairy, gluten, processed foods, excess sugar, alcohol)
- Introduction of anti-inflammatory additions (herbs, spices like turmeric or ginger)
- Weekly batch preparation of sinus-healthy snacks

For each day, tick off each habit achieved. At the week's end, review your tracker to spot patterns—consistently missed targets hint at where you may need to simplify routines or set reminders.

Table 10: Sample Habit Tracker Table for Sinusitis Diet Maintenance

Date	Monday	Tuesday	
Leafy Greens	✔	✔	
Vitamin C Food	✔		
Hydration Goal Met	✔		
No Trigger Foods	✔	✔	
Anti-Inflammatory Additions	✔		
Batch Snack Prep		✔	
Notes/Symptoms	Mild congestion AM	No congestion	

Reviewing this table allows you to troubleshoot adherence challenges and better understand which habits correlate with fewer symptoms.

Criteria for Safe Gradual Food Reintroductions and Monitoring for Rebound Symptoms

After consistently following an elimination diet and achieving symptom relief, many people are eager to diversify their diets without risking setbacks. The key is gradual and structured reintroduction. Effective maintenance requires you to test foods methodically, watching closely for even subtle sinus reactions.

Use these criteria when reintroducing foods:

- Only add one new food (or food group) at a time; wait at least 72 hours before adding another.
- Maintain a detailed log, noting quantity, time eaten, and any physical changes especially nasal congestion, sinus pressure, or changes in energy.
- If a mild reaction occurs (such as congestion or mild facial pressure), immediately return to your previous safe baseline and wait until all symptoms resolve before attempting another reintroduction.
- For more severe symptoms (intense headache, significant stuffiness, or prolonged fatigue), eliminate

the new food for at least 2–4 weeks before choosing whether to test it again.

This structured approach minimizes confusion around cause-and-effect and helps you determine your individual tolerance thresholds.

Social and Travel Survival Ruleset for Minimizing Accidental Exposures

Real-world eating rarely happens in carefully controlled environments. Restaurants, family gatherings, work events, and travel all pose accidental exposure risks. However, with the right mindset and protocols, you can enjoy social interactions while keeping your sinuses safe.

Consider implementing the following rules:

- Always review restaurant menus online beforehand, seeking options that align with your current phase of the Sinusitis Diet.
- Communicate clearly with hosts or servers mention specific ingredients that must be avoided, rather than general allergy requests.
- Carry sinus-friendly snacks (like fruit, unsalted nuts, homemade oat bars, or rice cakes) to avoid eating by default when safe options are limited.

- For travel, pack a mini "sinus-safe" kit: portable water bottle, hydrating teas, safe snack packs, antihistamine or saline spray if prescribed, and a symptom log.
- When unsure about food preparation (sauces, dressings, pre-made items), err on the side of caution and opt for the simplest dishes plain grilled meats or fish, steamed vegetables, salads without dressings you haven't prepared yourself.

Entering social settings with a plan lowers your chance of exposure and brings peace of mind whether you're at home or away.

Example Accountability Frameworks: Support Groups, Digital Tracking, or Professional Consultations

The journey toward sustained symptom control is made easier by reliable feedback and encouragement. Accountability can help keep dietary priorities top-of-mind, especially when initial motivation fades.

<u>Consider establishing one or more of these accountability systems:</u>

- Join an online or in-person support group focused on food sensitivities, allergy management, or sinus health. Regular check-ins provide both tips and moral support.
- Use a digital habit-tracking app tailored to dietary and symptom monitoring. Many allow sharing progress with friends, so you're not tracking alone.

- Set biweekly or monthly consultations with a nutritionist, health coach, or primary care provider. A professional can review your logs, troubleshoot obstacles, and help you adapt your plan as life circumstances change.
- Share your goals and progress with a trusted friend or family member who understands why your dietary vigilance matters. Ask them for encouragement and reminders, especially around family meals and social gatherings.

Having an "accountability anchor," whether high-tech or personal, supports your long-term consistency.

Long-Term Meal Planning Templates for Ongoing Sinus Health Stabilization

Without predictable, accessible meals that fit your Sinusitis Diet, it's easy to lapse into quick, convenience foods that may worsen symptoms. Organizing your grocery list and meals in advance is a cornerstone of long-term habit formation and relapse prevention.

A sample long-term meal planning approach includes:

1. ***Weekly "template menus"*** built around anti-inflammatory meals you know you tolerate well. For example:

   - *Breakfast*: Oatmeal with berries and pumpkin seeds, or smoothie with spinach, kiwi, and ginger.
   - *Lunch*: Grilled salmon salad with mixed greens, cucumber, and a lemon-olive oil vinaigrette.
   - *Snack*: Sliced apple with homemade sunflower seed butter.
   - *Dinner*: Roasted sweet potatoes, sautéed kale, and grilled chicken breast.
2. ***Plug pre-tested "modular"*** sides or proteins into each meal slot, rotating options to maintain variety while protecting from re-exposure to triggers.
3. ***Draft a shopping lis***t grouped by store section, streamlining weekly purchases (produce, whole grains, proteins, herbs, non-dairy alternatives).
4. ***Block time for weekly batch cooking*** or ingredient prep such as washing greens, chopping veggies, grilling proteins, and portioning snacks. Set reminders to restock critical sinus-friendly staples before running out.

A written meal plan not only saves time during busy weeks, it acts as a safety net, supporting adherence even during stressful periods or social disruptions.

Anticipating and Navigating Common Pitfalls

Long-term maintenance inevitably involves periods of lapse, temptation, or accident. Recognizing danger zones such as travel, celebrations, illness, or high-stress work periods lets you plan for extra self-monitoring.

If you notice recurring lapses:

- Revisit your tracker and accountability framework for gaps.
- Consider simplifying meal prep even further—batch-freeze safe meals, or rely on a short menu of quick-assembly dinners.
- Review your personal symptom timeline to reinforce why you started and what improves with adherence.

If symptoms persist despite ongoing careful diet, consult with a healthcare professional to rule out other contributing factors, review food logs for overlooked exposures, or consider a new cycle of structured elimination and reintroduction.

Successfully managing sinusitis through dietary changes is not just about short-term elimination phases. It requires turning new food choices, monitoring, and careful planning into lifelong habits. Leveraging habit trackers, introducing foods gradually, preparing social strategies, establishing accountability measures, and using templated meal planning all help set you up for steady and resilient sinus health. The result is greater confidence, fewer flares, and more freedom to enjoy life beyond the confines of sinus discomfort.

Sample Meal Plans for Sinusitis Relief

Finding daily meals that ease sinus discomfort can pose a persistent challenge, especially when transitioning to or maintaining a Sinusitis Diet. This chapter provides structured, actionable meal plans and resources that align with the Elimination and Substitution phases of the Sinusitis Diet 5-Step Plan.

The aim is to make meal preparation, ingredient selection, and nutritional analysis both systematic and practical so you can focus on healing rather than second-guessing every bite.

1-Week Meal Plan for Sinusitis Relief

Below is a sample 7-day meal plan specifically crafted to support sinus health. This plan emphasizes anti-inflammatory ingredients, avoids common triggers (such as dairy, gluten, refined sugars, and processed foods), and incorporates hydrating and immunity-supportive nutrients. Where relevant, suitable ingredient substitutions ensure the plan remains accessible to those with additional allergies or dietary restrictions.

Day 1

- ***Breakfast***: Warm oatmeal with blueberries, chia seeds, and a sprinkle of cinnamon (substitute oat milk for nut intolerance)
- ***Snack***: Sliced cucumber and carrot sticks with hummus dip
- ***Lunch***: Quinoa salad with roasted sweet potato, fresh spinach, chickpeas, and lemon-olive oil dressing
- ***Snack***: An apple with pumpkin seeds Dinner: Grilled salmon with steamed broccoli and brown rice

Day 2

- ***Breakfast***: Smoothie with spinach, kiwi, pineapple, and unsweetened coconut milk
- ***Snack***: Rice cakes topped with mashed avocado and a squeeze of lemon
- ***Lunch***: Turkey lettuce wraps with cucumber, bell pepper, and shredded carrot
- ***Snack***: Pear slices and a handful of sunflower seeds Dinner: Stir-fried tofu with mixed veggies (broccoli, snow peas, red pepper) and gluten-free tamari, served with millet

Day 3

- ***Breakfast***: Overnight oats with strawberries, flaxseed, and unsweetened almond milk
- ***Snack***: Fresh orange segments
- ***Lunch***: Grilled chicken breast over arugula, cherry tomatoes, and beet ribbons
- ***Snack***: Homemade trail mix (pumpkin seeds, unsweetened coconut flakes, dried cranberries)
- ***Dinner***: Baked cod with roasted fennel and quinoa tabbouleh (swap cod with tempeh for plant-based)

Day 4

- ***Breakfast***: Brown rice cakes with almond butter and sliced banana
- ***Snack***: Celery sticks with sunflower seed butter
- ***Lunch***: Lentil soup with carrots, celery, and bay leaf (ensure gluten-free broth)
- ***Snack***: Diced mango with lime
- ***Dinner***: Baked sweet potato with sautéed kale and garlic, topped with toasted pepitas

Day 5

- ***Breakfast***: Dairy-free chia pudding with raspberries and shredded coconut
- ***Snack***: Bell pepper strips with guacamole
- ***Lunch***: Chickpea and spinach curry with brown basmati rice

- ***Snack***: Pineapple chunks with fresh mint
- ***Dinner***: Baked turkey breast, quinoa pilaf with parsley and lemon zest, steamed green beans

Day 6

- ***Breakfast***: Millet porridge with diced apple, cinnamon, and coconut cream
- ***Snack***: Fresh grapes
- ***Lunch***: Roasted cauliflower and carrot salad with tahini dressing
- ***Snack***: Rice crackers with mashed avocado and tomato slices
- ***Dinner***: Grilled tilapia with sautéed zucchini and wild rice (tilapia can be swapped with chickpea patties for vegan)

Day 7

- ***Breakfast***: Green smoothie (kale, cucumber, pear, ginger, and coconut water)
- ***Snack***: Unsweetened applesauce with cinnamon
- ***Lunch***: Quinoa and bean bowl with roasted red peppers, spinach, and cumin-lime dressing

- ***Snack***: Steamed edamame
- ***Dinner***: Grilled chicken kebabs with bell peppers and onions, served with herbed millet salad

Each day, the plan prioritizes whole, minimally processed foods and includes options for plant-based or animal protein sources, ensuring flexibility for personal preferences and dietary needs.

Sinus-Healthy Recipe Index with Preparation Instructions

Oatmeal with Blueberries and Chia Seeds

Ingredients:

- ½ cup gluten-free rolled oats
- 1 cup oat milk or almond milk
- ¼ cup fresh or frozen blueberries
- 1 tablespoon chia seeds
- ½ teaspoon ground cinnamon

Instructions:

1. In a small saucepan, combine the gluten-free rolled oats and your choice of oat milk or almond milk.
2. Place the saucepan over medium heat and bring the mixture to a gentle simmer, stirring occasionally to prevent sticking.
3. Allow the oats to cook for about 5 minutes, or until they have absorbed most of the liquid and reached your desired consistency.
4. Add the blueberries, chia seeds, and ground cinnamon to the saucepan. Stir well to evenly distribute the ingredients.

5. Continue to cook for an additional 1-2 minutes, until the blueberries are warmed through and the chia seeds have begun to thicken the oatmeal.
6. Remove from heat and let the oatmeal sit for a minute to cool slightly and thicken further.
7. Serve the oatmeal warm. Optionally, garnish with extra blueberries or a drizzle of maple syrup if desired.

Quinoa Salad with Roasted Sweet Potato

Ingredients:

- 1 sweet potato, diced
- Olive oil (for roasting)
- 1 cup cooked quinoa
- 1 cup fresh spinach
- ½ cup chickpeas (canned or cooked)
- 2 tablespoons lemon-olive oil dressing

Instructions:

1. Preheat the oven to 400°F (200°C).
2. Toss the diced sweet potato with olive oil, then spread it on a baking sheet.
3. Roast the sweet potato in the oven for 25 minutes, or until tender and lightly browned.
4. In a large bowl, combine the roasted sweet potato, cooked quinoa, fresh spinach, and chickpeas.
5. Drizzle the lemon-olive oil dressing over the salad.
6. Toss everything together until well combined.
7. Serve immediately.

Turkey Lettuce Wraps

Ingredients:

- Crisp romaine leaves
- ½ cup cooked turkey breast, shredded
- Sliced cucumber
- Sliced bell pepper
- Sliced carrot
- Olive oil
- Fresh herbs

Instructions:

1. Arrange romaine leaves on a plate.
2. Fill each leaf with shredded turkey, cucumber, bell pepper, and carrot.
3. Drizzle with olive oil and sprinkle with fresh herbs.
4. Serve immediately.

Lentil Soup with Carrots and Celery

Ingredients:

- 1 onion, chopped
- 2 carrots, chopped
- 2 celery stalks, chopped
- Olive oil
- 1 cup brown lentils, rinsed
- 4 cups vegetable broth
- 1 bay leaf
- Salt and pepper, to taste

Instructions:

1. Sauté onion, carrots, and celery in olive oil in a large pot until soft.
2. Add rinsed lentils, vegetable broth, and bay leaf.
3. Simmer for 30 minutes.
4. Season with salt and pepper to taste.
5. Remove bay leaf before serving.

Chickpea and Spinach Curry

Ingredients:

- 1 onion, diced
- Olive oil
- 1 clove garlic, minced
- 1 teaspoon turmeric
- 1 teaspoon cumin
- 1 can chickpeas, rinsed
- 3 cups fresh spinach
- 1 can coconut milk
- Cooked rice, for serving

Instructions:

1. Sauté diced onion in olive oil in a large pan.
2. Add minced garlic, turmeric, and cumin; cook until fragrant.
3. Add chickpeas and spinach; stir to combine.
4. Pour in coconut milk and simmer for 10 minutes.
5. Serve hot with rice.

Grilled Chicken Kebabs

Ingredients:

- Chicken breast, cut into chunks
- Bell pepper, cut into chunks
- Onion, cut into chunks
- Olive oil
- Mixed herbs (such as oregano, thyme, or rosemary)

Instructions:

1. Alternate pieces of chicken breast, bell pepper, and onion on skewers.
2. Brush the assembled skewers with olive oil.
3. Season with mixed herbs.
4. Grill for 10–12 minutes, turning occasionally, until the chicken is cooked through.

Avocado and Tomato Toast

Ingredients:

- 1 slice gluten-free bread
- ½ avocado, sliced
- ¼ cup cherry tomatoes, halved
- Salt and pepper, to taste
- Olive oil

Instructions:

1. Toast the gluten-free bread.
2. Top with sliced avocado and halved cherry tomatoes.
3. Sprinkle with salt and pepper.
4. Drizzle with olive oil and serve immediately.

Broccoli and White Bean Stir-Fry

Ingredients:

- 2 cups broccoli florets
- Olive oil
- 1 can white beans, drained
- 1 teaspoon grated ginger
- 2 tablespoons low-sodium tamari

Instructions:

1. Sauté broccoli florets in olive oil for 5 minutes over medium heat.
2. Add drained white beans, grated ginger, and tamari.
3. Cook for 2–3 more minutes, stirring gently.
4. Serve hot.

Baked Salmon with Lemon and Dill

Ingredients:

- 4-ounce salmon fillet
- Lemon slices
- Fresh dill

Instructions:

1. Place the salmon fillet on a baking tray.
2. Top with lemon slices and fresh dill.
3. Bake at 375°F (190°C) for 15–18 minutes, or until cooked through.

Sweet Potato and Black Bean Tacos

Ingredients:

- 1 sweet potato, diced
- ½ cup black beans
- Corn tortillas
- Shredded lettuce
- Salsa

Instructions:

1. Preheat oven to 400°F (200°C).
2. Roast the diced sweet potato for 25 minutes.
3. Fill corn tortillas with roasted sweet potato, black beans, shredded lettuce, and salsa.

Cucumber and Mint Smoothie

Ingredients:

- 1 cucumber, peeled
- 1 cup spinach
- ½ cup coconut water
- 1 tablespoon fresh mint
- ½ green apple

Instructions:

1. Blend the peeled cucumber, spinach, coconut water, fresh mint, and green apple until smooth.
2. Serve chilled.

Eggplant and Chickpea Stew

Ingredients:

- 1 eggplant, diced
- 1 onion, chopped
- Olive oil
- 1 can tomatoes
- 1 can chickpeas
- 1 teaspoon smoked paprika

Instructions:

1. Sauté diced eggplant and chopped onion in olive oil until tender.
2. Add canned tomatoes, chickpeas, and smoked paprika.
3. Simmer for 20 minutes.

Brown Rice and Veggie Bowl

Ingredients:

- 1 cup brown rice
- Steamed broccoli
- Steamed carrots
- Steamed snap peas
- Tahini-lemon sauce
- Sesame seeds

Instructions:

1. Cook 1 cup brown rice according to package instructions.
2. Top with steamed broccoli, carrots, and snap peas.
3. Drizzle with tahini-lemon sauce and sprinkle with sesame seeds.

Apple Cinnamon Chia Pudding

Ingredients:

- 3 tablespoons chia seeds
- 1 cup almond milk
- ½ grated apple
- ½ teaspoon cinnamon

Instructions:

1. Mix chia seeds, almond milk, grated apple, and cinnamon in a bowl or jar.
2. Refrigerate overnight.
3. Serve chilled.

Carrot and Ginger Soup

Ingredients:

- 1 onion, chopped
- 4 carrots, chopped
- Olive oil
- 1 teaspoon grated ginger
- 3 cups vegetable broth
- Salt and pepper (to taste)

Instructions:

1. Sauté chopped onion and carrots in olive oil until softened.
2. Add grated ginger and cook for 1 minute.
3. Pour in vegetable broth and simmer for 20 minutes.
4. Blend the soup until smooth.
5. Season with salt and pepper to taste.

Stuffed Bell Peppers with Quinoa

Ingredients:

- 2 bell peppers
- 1 cup cooked quinoa
- ½ cup black beans
- ¼ cup corn

Instructions:

1. Cut the tops off bell peppers and remove seeds.
2. Mix cooked quinoa, black beans, and corn in a bowl.
3. Fill peppers with the mixture.
4. Place in a baking dish and bake at 375°F (190°C) for 30 minutes.

Zucchini Noodles with Pesto

Ingredients:

- 2 zucchinis
- 2 tablespoons dairy-free pesto
- ½ cup cherry tomatoes, halved

Instructions:

1. Spiralize the zucchinis to make noodles.
2. Toss noodles with dairy-free pesto and cherry tomatoes.
3. Serve chilled or lightly warmed.

Tuna and White Bean Salad

Ingredients:

- 1 can tuna, drained
- 1 can white beans, drained
- ¼ cup diced celery
- 2 tablespoons olive oil
- Juice of ½ lemon

Greens, for serving

Instructions:

1. Mix tuna, white beans, diced celery, olive oil, and lemon juice in a bowl.
2. Serve over greens.

Roasted Cauliflower with Turmeric

Ingredients:

- 2 cups cauliflower florets
- 1 tablespoon olive oil
- 1 teaspoon turmeric

Instructions:

1. Preheat oven to 425°F (220°C).
2. Toss cauliflower florets with olive oil and turmeric.
3. Spread on a baking sheet and roast for 20–25 minutes.

Berry and Spinach Yogurt Parfait

Ingredients:

- 1 cup dairy-free yogurt (such as oat, almond, or rice milk-based)
- 1 cup mixed berries
- ½ cup fresh spinach, chopped
- 1 tablespoon chia seeds

Instructions:

1. In a glass, layer ½ cup of dairy-free yogurt.
2. Add ½ cup of mixed berries on top of the yogurt.
3. Sprinkle ¼ cup of chopped fresh spinach over the berries.
4. Repeat the layers with the remaining yogurt, berries, and spinach.
5. Top the parfait with chia seeds before serving.

Ingredient Substitutions:

- Use rice milk-based yogurt instead of oat or almond for nut avoidance.
- Substitute tofu, tempeh, or bean-based patties in place of animal proteins in other recipes.
- Opt for gluten-free oats and bread products to accommodate gluten sensitivities.

These recipes are designed for practical use; preparations can be scaled and ingredients swapped according to your current safe food list.

Shopping List Aligned with Elimination and Substitution Phases

This list fits the recommended dietary boundaries for sinus relief, covering elimination (avoiding triggers) and substitution (healthy replacements).

- ***Produce***: Spinach, kale, arugula, broccoli, carrots, celery, sweet potatoes, tomatoes, zucchini, cucumber, bell peppers, onions, garlic, fennel, green beans, mango, banana, apple, pear, pineapple, blueberries, raspberries, strawberries, grapes, oranges, lemon, lime, fresh herbs (parsley, mint)
- ***Whole Grains and Legumes***: Gluten-free oats, millet, brown/wild rice, quinoa, brown basmati rice, chickpeas, lentils, black beans, edamame

- ***Protein***: Chicken breast, turkey, salmon, tilapia, cod, tofu, tempeh, pumpkin seeds, sunflower seeds, nut/seed butters (almond, sunflower), unsalted nuts (if tolerated)
- ***Healthy Fats***: Olive oil, coconut oil, tahini, unsweetened coconut
- ***Non-Dairy Alternatives***: Oat milk, almond milk, coconut milk, rice milk
- ***Snacks***: Rice cakes, rice crackers, unsweetened applesauce, dried fruit (in moderation), homemade trail mix (no added sugar)
- ***Pantry Staples***: Gluten-free broth, turmeric, cumin, cinnamon, black pepper, bay leaf

This well-structured shopping list reduces time in the store and ensures your kitchen is always stocked for sinus-friendly meal preparation.

Rotating Pantry Staples Table for Flexibility and Flavor

Keep your pantry versatile and meals exciting by rotating these staples weekly:

Table 11: Rotating Pantry Staples Table

Pantry Staple	Substitution Options	Tips for Variety
Gluten-free oats	Brown rice, millet	Rotate for hot/cold breakfasts
Quinoa	Wild rice, buckwheat	Use as salads, pilafs
Canned	Lentils, black beans	For soups, stews,

chickpeas		or dips
Olive oil	Coconut oil, avocado oil	Vary dressings & cooking
Unsweetened coconut	Chia seeds, flaxseeds	Add to porridge, pudding
Nut butters	Sunflower seed butter	Adjust for allergies

This approach keeps meals interesting while supporting adherence to anti-inflammatory, sinus-safe eating routines.

Nutritional Analysis Grid

Optimal sinus support requires both avoidance of triggers and focus on nutrients that boost immunity, reduce inflammation, and promote clear airways. Below, meals are matched to key nutrients important for sinusitis relief:

Table 12: Nutritional Analysis Grid

Meal	Key Nutrients	Symptom Management Role
Oatmeal with blueberries	Fiber, vitamin C, antioxidants	Mucus thinning, immune support
Grilled salmon with greens	Omega-3s, vitamin D, magnesium	Anti-inflammatory, tissue repair
Spinach-kiwi smoothie	Vitamin C, folate, potassium	Immunity, reduced swelling
Lentil soup	Plant protein, B vitamins, iron	Energy, repair, mucus clearance
Chickpea & spinach curry	Plant protein, iron, vitamin E	Reduces reactive cycles, sustains energy
Roasted sweet potato	Beta-carotene, potassium, fiber	Improves barrier function
Turkey lettuce wraps	Lean protein, B vitamins, zinc	Supports healing, mucosal barrier

This grid allows you to select and rotate meals according to your individual needs—ensuring nutritional diversity while supporting sinus wellness goals.

Adopting a structured, sinus-friendly meal plan can make a significant difference in managing sinusitis symptoms and supporting overall well-being. With practical recipes, flexible ingredient substitutions, and a clear shopping guide, this chapter helps simplify daily food choices while keeping meals flavorful and nourishing. The rotating pantry staples and nutritional analysis grid make it easy to maintain variety and meet essential nutrient needs. Consistent use of these strategies empowers you to focus on healing and enjoying food without the stress of dietary guesswork.

Troubleshooting and Common Challenges

Successfully managing sinusitis through dietary changes can be rewarding, but it is not always a straightforward path. Even after diligently following the Sinusitis Diet 5-Step Plan, some individuals face stubborn symptoms, unexpected setbacks, or confusing patterns of improvement and flare-up. This chapter is designed to provide practical troubleshooting tools, help you identify persistent or overlooked obstacles, and clarify when to escalate to professional care.

Diagnostic Flowchart for Persistent Symptoms Despite Dietary Changes

If your sinusitis symptoms continue or even worsen despite making the recommended dietary modifications, it is crucial to approach troubleshooting in a systematic and thorough way. The following diagnostic flowchart outlines a step-by-step process to help you reassess your situation and identify potential reasons for your persistent symptoms:

1. **Confirm Adherence to Dietary Recommendations**

   Begin by carefully evaluating whether you are strictly following the elimination and substitution guidelines provided. Examine every aspect of your diet, paying close attention to packaged foods, restaurant meals, and beverages, as these can often contain hidden sources of common trigger foods such as dairy, gluten, or soy. Even trace amounts of these ingredients sometimes present due to cross-contamination—can be enough to provoke symptoms and undermine your progress.

2. **Revisit Food and Symptom Logs**

   Next, review your food and symptom journal in detail. Note any episodes of symptom flare-ups and cross-reference these with foods recently introduced or consumed accidentally. Look for patterns that might reveal subtle triggers. Pay particular attention to any new foods, spices, or preparation methods, as these may have introduced unexpected allergens or irritants.

3. **Rule Out Cross-Reactions**

   Some foods can cause reactions due to cross-reactivity, especially if you have a history of pollen allergies such as birch, ragweed, or grass. For example, individuals with birch pollen allergies may react to apples, carrots, or hazelnuts. Evaluate whether exposure to related foods, spices, or even herbal teas could be contributing to your ongoing symptoms.

4. **Evaluate Environmental Factors**

   Remember, diet is just one factor influencing sinus health. Environmental allergens including dust mites, pollen, mold, animal dander as well as exposure to strong chemicals, fragrances, cigarette smoke, or abrupt weather changes, can all sustain or worsen sinus symptoms. Consider whether recent changes in your environment or routines could be playing a role.

5. **Assess Overall Hydration and Anti-Inflammatory Support**

   Ensure that you are maintaining optimal hydration throughout the day and consuming a diet rich in anti-inflammatory foods such as leafy greens, berries, fatty fish, and healthy fats. Inadequate fluid intake or insufficient phytonutrients can impede your recovery and exacerbate inflammation .

6. **Consider Structural or Medical Causes**

   If symptoms persist despite careful dietary and environmental management, consult a healthcare professional to investigate structural or underlying medical causes. Issues such as a deviated septum, nasal polyps, chronic infections, or immune deficiencies may require targeted medical interventions. Further diagnostic testing may be necessary to rule out these possibilities and develop an appropriate treatment plan.

If you reach the final step with ongoing symptoms after systematically eliminating each factor above, it's time to involve healthcare professionals for specialized evaluation.

Checklist for Reviewing Overlooked Triggers, Cross-Reactivity, and Environmental Factors

To leave no stone unturned, use this troubleshooting checklist to systematically review your potential exposures:

- Have you checked ingredient lists for all processed foods, sauces, dressings, and snacks?
- Are you regularly consuming any foods that could share cross-reactive proteins with environmental allergens (e.g., apple and birch pollen, melon and ragweed)?
- Is your kitchen free from common hidden sources of your personal triggers (for example, wheat-based thickeners, casein in processed meats, or soy in seasoning blends)?
- Are housemates, family members, or visitors introducing allergens through shared cookware, crumbs, or airborne particles?

- Are you using only hypoallergenic, fragrance-free household cleaners and laundry products?
- Do seasonal pollen counts or air quality alerts coincide with your symptom spikes?
- Have you recently traveled, eaten at restaurants, or attended gatherings where control over food preparation was limited?
- Are you maintaining consistent hydration, especially on travel or high-activity days?
- Are you exposed to cigarette smoke, incense, or environmental pollutants at home or work?

Carefully address each point in the checklist, as even a minor overlooked element can trigger breakthrough symptoms.

Examples of Common Failure Modes and Resolution Tactics

Individuals managing sinusitis through dietary strategies often encounter various failure modes that can undermine their efforts. Identifying these challenges early and implementing targeted solutions is key for sustained symptom control. Here are some common pitfalls and actionable tactics to address them:

1. **Hidden or Accidental Exposure**

   Even the most vigilant individuals can unknowingly consume hidden sources of gluten, dairy, or other dietary triggers. These ingredients can lurk in processed foods under ambiguous terms such as "natural flavors," "casein" in deli meats, or even in condiments like soy sauce, which often contains gluten.

Resolution: Practice being a label detective. Carefully read ingredient lists, learn common alternate names for your triggers, and, when in doubt, reach out to manufacturers for clarification. When possible, opt for single-ingredient or minimally processed foods to reduce the risk of accidental exposure.

2. **Cumulative Effects of Minor Triggers**

   While a single small exposure to a trigger might not lead to immediate symptoms, repeated minor exposures can have a cumulative effect. This can result in a delayed or seemingly random flare-up of sinus symptoms, making it difficult to pinpoint the cause.

   Resolution: Maintain a detailed food and symptom diary to track potential patterns. If you suspect cumulative effects, consider returning to a stricter elimination phase for one to two weeks to "reset" your symptom baseline. This can help you identify and avoid subtle triggers more effectively.

3. **Underestimating Cross-Reactivity**

   Certain foods, such as celery, nuts, or specific spices, may cross-react with environmental allergens (like pollen or dust mites), potentially worsening sinusitis symptoms.

   Resolution: Cross-reference your known environmental allergies with established cross-reactivity food charts. During peak allergy seasons, consider eliminating these foods temporarily to assess their impact on your symptoms.

4. **Lax Hydration and Mucus Thinning**

   Adequate hydration is crucial for thinning mucus and reducing congestion, yet it is often neglected. Even mild dehydration can lead to thicker mucus, making sinus symptoms worse.

   Resolution: Use alarms, hydration tracking apps, or pre-filled water bottles to ensure you're consistently meeting your daily fluid needs. Aim for clear or lightly tinted urine as a sign of good hydration.

5. **Environmental Sabotage**

   Persistent exposure to indoor irritants such as mold, pet dander, or smoke can negate dietary improvements and perpetuate sinus inflammation.

Resolution: Invest in air purifiers with HEPA filters, clean regularly with HEPA vacuums, keep windows closed on high pollen days, and address known sources of household irritants promptly.

6. **Supplement or Medication Interactions**

   Supplements or medications taken for sinus support may inadvertently contain hidden triggers (for example, dairy-derived capsules) or may interact with other medications, potentially worsening symptoms.

   Resolution: Consult with your healthcare provider or pharmacist before starting any new supplement. Check ingredient lists carefully, and ask specifically about allergen-free formulations if you are sensitive to certain compounds.

Awareness of these common failure modes, combined with proactive use of these resolution tactics, allows individuals managing sinusitis through diet to increase their chances of long-term success and reduce the risk of unexpected setbacks.

Referral Criteria: When to Seek Medical or Dietary Specialist Support

While dietary strategies can dramatically improve sinus health in many cases, there are clear situations where professional input is essential:

- Persistent or worsening symptoms after diligent adherence to elimination and substitution protocols
- Symptoms suggesting infection, such as fever, severe facial pain, vision changes, or colored nasal discharge
- Signs of allergic reactions (swelling, hives, difficulty breathing) after food or environmental exposures
- Complex dietary needs (multiple allergies, nutritional deficiencies, or malnutrition risk)
- Difficulty designing a sustainable, balanced meal plan amid extensive food restrictions
- Severe impact on daily living or mood from chronic sinus issues

In these scenarios, reach out to a primary care provider first for evaluation. Referral to an allergist, otolaryngologist (ENT), or registered dietitian may be recommended for targeted testing and management.

Emergency Action Protocol for Severe or Sudden Onset Sinus Symptoms

Although sinusitis most often builds gradually, certain signs require immediate action:

- Sudden, severe headache associated with fever, confusion, or neck stiffness
- Swelling of eyes or face, or vision changes
- Severe, unrelenting facial pain or inability to breathe comfortably through both nostrils

- Persistent vomiting, dehydration, or inability to keep down fluids
- Rapid onset of allergic reaction, including throat tightness, trouble swallowing, or wheezing

If any of these develop, seek urgent medical attention. In the interim, stop all suspected foods, hydrate with clear fluids if possible, and clarify your history and recent exposures for healthcare providers.

Troubleshooting sinusitis with dietary strategies is a dynamic process. By systematically reviewing your exposure, maintaining rigorous records, and recognizing when to seek specialized help, you can significantly improve your chances of long-term sinus relief.

Conclusion

As you reach the end of the Sinusitis Diet Guide, it's clear that managing sinus congestion and irritation requires ongoing attention and flexibility. Implementing dietary changes using the 5-Step Plan is only the start; maintaining and refining those strategies can lead to lasting symptom relief, especially during allergy seasons or times of increased environmental triggers. Here, we'll review practical next steps, key factors for sustained improvement, and how to fully integrate dietary practices into your broader sinus wellness routine.

Practical next steps for continued improvement involve regular symptom monitoring and active engagement with your daily nutrition choices. Continue logging your meals and any associated symptoms, paying careful attention to even minor flare-ups. This practice helps you catch delayed reactions, accidental exposures, or emerging sensitivities as your body and environment change over time. If you notice new symptoms or patterns, don't hesitate to repeat elimination steps or tighten your substitution strategies. Keeping a detailed symptom-tracker ensures you have data on which foods or conditions are most reliably linked to congestion, pressure, or fatigue.

Long-term success hinges on several critical factors, including dietary consistency, the ability to adapt, and the willingness to re-evaluate your plan as circumstances evolve. Key influences include seasonal allergy fluctuations, travel or social eating conditions, and any new medical diagnoses. Learning to adapt your meal plans by swapping in safe, anti-inflammatory foods or temporarily avoiding additional risk items during peak allergy months will help you stay ahead of new triggers.

It is also essential to assess your hydration status regularly and retain a pantry stocked with supportive, nutrient-focused staples to avoid lapses into high-risk, processed foods. When dining out or attending social events, proactive communication about your needs and careful menu review can minimize accidental exposures and maintain your progress.

Integrating dietary strategies with your sinus wellness routines means looking beyond a "food only" focus. Sinus health thrives on synergy between diet, environmental management, and healthy lifestyle behaviors. Continue optimizing your anti-inflammatory food choices while maintaining strict avoidance of your individual triggers.

Pair dietary changes with effective allergen avoidance at home, such as using air purifiers, cleaning with hypoallergenic products, and controlling pollen or dust exposures. Regular moderate exercise and stress management also support immune balance and overall wellness, further enhancing the effects of your dietary efforts.

It is important to view the Sinusitis Diet Plan as a dynamic, adaptable toolkit. Be willing to refine your strategies, experiment with new recipes, and involve healthcare professionals when necessary for guidance or troubleshooting. If you experience setbacks, review your logs, environmental exposures, and substitution choices before making adjustments. And above all, celebrate your progress—no matter the pace. Every step toward personalized, balanced nutrition is a step toward clearer breathing and improved quality of life.

FAQs

Which foods are most likely to trigger sinus congestion during allergy season?

Certain foods often worsen sinus congestion, particularly during allergy season. Dairy products: like milk, cheese, and cream are among the top triggers, as they can increase mucus production. Wheat and gluten-containing foods (bread, pasta, baked goods) are also common triggers, potentially causing inflammation or mild allergic reactions in sensitive people. Refined sugars should be limited as they promote inflammation and can intensify sinus discomfort.

Processed foods, high in additives and sodium, may increase water retention and swelling in mucous membranes, worsening sinus blockage. Alcohol, especially beer and wine, can dehydrate and irritate mucosal tissues, increasing congestion during allergy peaks. Triggers can vary, so tracking symptoms and identifying personal sensitivities is key, but these foods are generally the highest priority for elimination.

How quickly should I expect to see improvements after changing my diet?

Improvement timelines vary. Some people notice relief, like less congestion or easier breathing within a few days of removing a dietary irritant, especially if it was a regular part of their diet. For others, especially those with chronic sinusitis, benefits may appear after two to four weeks.

Consistency is important to allow the body to reduce inflammation. If no meaningful changes are noticed after four weeks of strict adherence, reassess possible overlooked triggers or consult a healthcare provider. During allergy season, improvements may take longer due to increased environmental factors.

Can dietary changes completely eliminate the need for sinus medication?

For some, especially those with diet-responsive sinusitis, comprehensive dietary changes can significantly reduce or even eliminate the need for sinus medications. However, not everyone will achieve medication independence. Those with more severe sinus issues or other ongoing risk factors may still need medications alongside dietary changes.

The Sinusitis Diet Guide emphasizes that while food-based management is powerful, you should always consult a healthcare professional before changing prescribed medications. For many, improved dietary habits can mean lower doses or less frequent medication use, but dietary strategies are a complement, not a replacement, for medical care when needed.

What should I do if I react to a food that is not a common sinus trigger?

Everyone's sensitivities are unique. If you react to an uncommon food, document it in your food journal. Remove the food for at least two weeks and monitor symptoms. If you improve, try reintroducing it on a day when you feel well and allergens are low. If the reaction returns, consider that food a personal trigger and avoid it. Less common reactions can be due to cross-reactivity, intolerance, or hidden additives, so check labels carefully and keep detailed records.

How can I balance my diet if I have multiple food sensitivities and require eliminations?

Managing multiple eliminations can be challenging, but a balanced diet is possible with planning. Focus on whole, unprocessed foods that are naturally low in common triggers, such as fresh fruits and vegetables, lean poultry or fish, and gluten- and dairy-free grains like rice or quinoa.

Use substitution checklists and meal planning tools to find safe alternatives like plant-based milks or gluten-free products. Rotate foods to prevent new sensitivities, seek variety, and use your symptom tracker to spot issues. If needed, consult a registered dietitian experienced with food allergies and sinusitis to ensure nutritional adequacy.

Are supplements recommended as part of the Sinusitis Diet Plan?

The Sinusitis Diet Guide focuses on whole-food strategies, but supplements can help if dietary restrictions limit essential nutrients or if deficiencies are diagnosed. Key nutrients for sinus and immune health include vitamin C, zinc, and quercetin, which are best obtained from a colorful, varied diet.

Hydration with herbal teas and broths is also beneficial. Consult your healthcare provider before starting supplements, as they may interact with medications or other conditions. Supplements should support, not replace, a varied diet.

If my symptoms do not improve, should I see an allergist or nutritionist next?

If you've followed the guide and still have symptoms, the next step depends on your situation. If your history suggests allergies like seasonal patterns or multiple sensitivities consult an allergist for testing and treatment. If your symptoms seem more tied to food or you struggle with dietary adjustments, a nutritionist or registered dietitian can help refine your meal plan. Sometimes, working with both professionals offers the best results, as allergists address immune triggers and dietitians optimize nutrition. Always keep your primary healthcare provider informed.

References and Helpful Links

Fokkens, W., Lund, V., Hopkins, C. et al.. European Position Paper on Rhinosinusitis and Nasal Polyps 2020. https://doi.org/10.4193/rhin20.600

Frosh, A., Cruz, C., Wellsted, D., & Stephens, J.. Effect of a dairy diet on nasopharyngeal mucus secretion. The Laryngoscope, 129(1), 13-17... 20. Accessed February 12, 2026. https://onlinelibrary.wiley.com/doi/abs/10.1002/lary.27287

Ma, X. Nan, F., Liang, H. et al.. Excessive intake of sugar: An accomplice of inflammation. Frontiers in Immunology. doi:10./fimmu.81. 20. Accessed February 12, 2026. https://www.frontiersin.org/articles/10.3389/fimmu.2022.988481/full

Deng, Y., Wang, C., Shen, S., Yang, X., Lou, H., & Zhang, L.. Effects of acute alcohol intake on nasal patency. American Journal of Rhinology & Allergy, 36(3), 330-338... 2022. Accessed February 12, 2026. https://journals.sagepub.com/doi/abs/10.1177/19458924211062322

Wüthrich, B. Schmid, A., Walther, B. et al.. Milk Consumption Does Not Lead to Mucus Production or Occurrence of Asthma. Journal of the American College of Nutrition. doi:10./. 20. Accessed February 12, 2026. https://www.tandfonline.com/doi/abs/10.1080/07315724.2005.10719503

Yonkers, A. J. (1992). Sinusitis—inspecting the causes and treatment. Ear, nose & throat journal, 71(6), 258-262. 1992. Accessed February 12, 2026.
https://journals.sagepub.com/doi/abs/10.1177/014556139207100602

Linder, J. Atlas, S.. Health-related quality of life in patients with sinusitis. Current Allergy and Asthma Reports. doi:10./s2-004--1. 20. Accessed February 12, 2026.
https://link.springer.com/article/10.1007/s11882-004-0017-1

www.ingramcontent.com/pod-product-compliance
Lightning Source LLC
LaVergne TN
LVHW020234210926
848481LV00016B/2189